What A Melon

From the motherland to Your Mouth

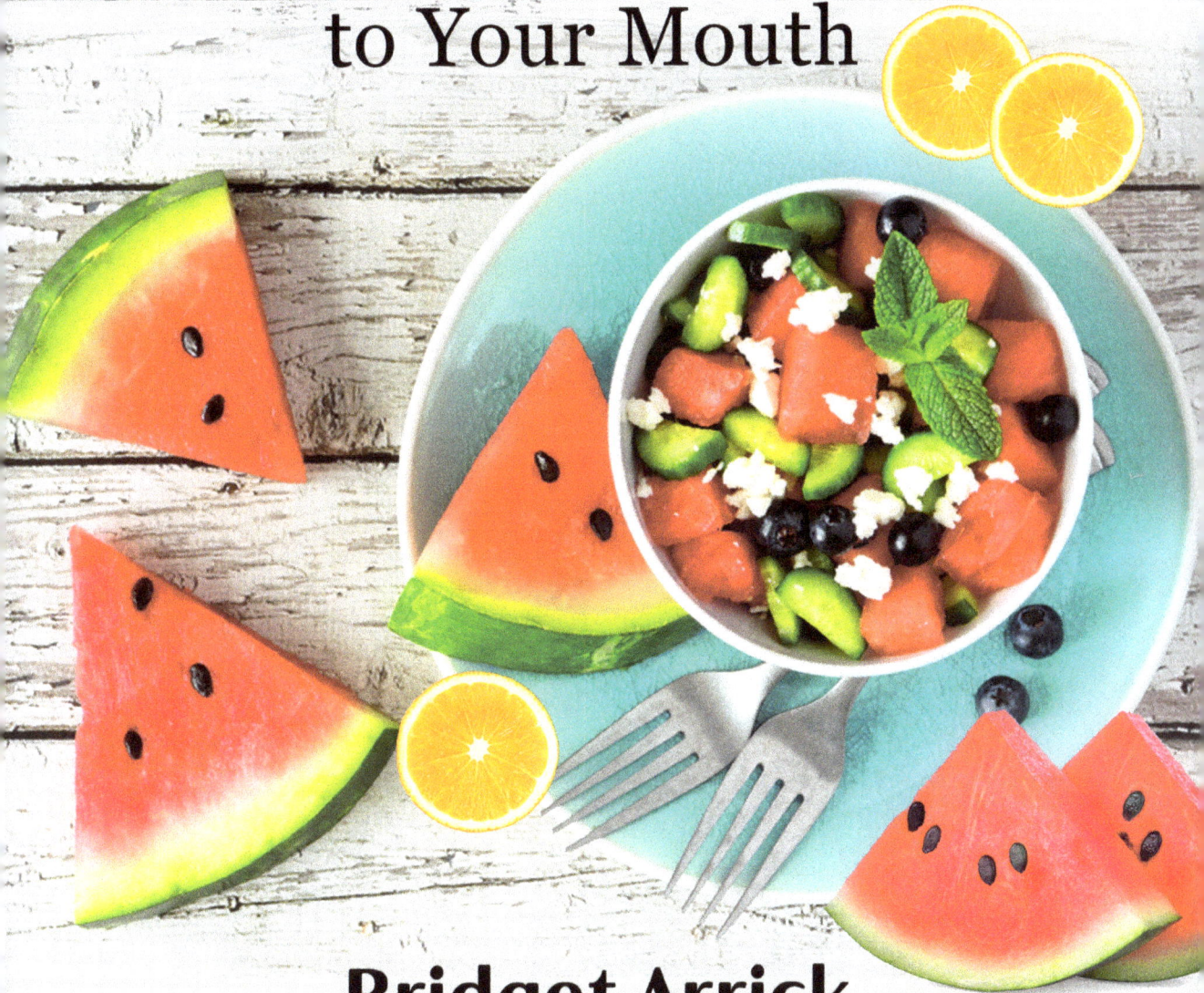

Bridget Arrick

aka Author Vacation Girlfriend

What A Melon: From the the Motherland to Your Mouth

A Juicy Celebration of Culture, Health & Sweet Living

Copyright © 2025 Bridget Arrick aka Vacation Girlfriend

Catalog-in-Publication Data is on file with the the Library of Congress

For permission requests, contact the publisher at:

authorvacationgirlfriend@gmail.com

Published By : Author Vacation Girlfriend LLC,
Harrington DE, 19952

Printed in the United States of America.
First Edition 2025

ISBN: 979-8-9987170-4-8

What A Melon

From the Motherland to Your Mouth

A Juicy Celebration of Culture, Health & Sweet Living

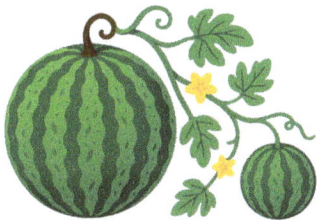

What A Melon: From the Motherland to Your Mouth

A Juicy Celebration of Culture, Health & Sweet Living

The Sweetest Story Never Told

Before watermelon was a picnic icon or a summer snack it was royalty in the sands of Africa. Yes, royalty. Carved into the walls of ancient tombs in Nubia and Egypt, watermelon has long symbolized abundance, hydration, and healing. But somewhere along the journey through colonization, commodification, and cultural erasure this juicy gem lost her crown.

This book is a reclaiming.

"What A Melon" is more than a health guide. It's a celebration of history, flavor, wellness, and joy. Whether you eat it by the wedge, blend it in a smoothie, or grill it with a little spice and sass, watermelon is for the culture and the cure. We're bringing it all back: seeded varieties, vibrant flesh colors, recipes that nourish, and ancestral practices that heal.

So welcome to the juiciest book you've ever opened. From rind to shine this one's for you

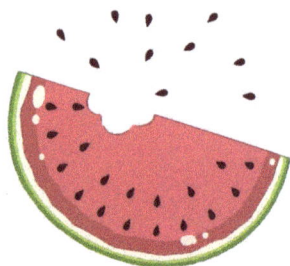

Table of Contents

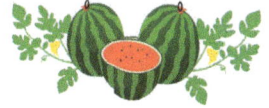

Introduction
The Sweetest Story Ever Told

Chapter 1: The African Origins of Watermelon

Before watermelon became a symbol of summer in the U.S., it was revered in Africa as a divine fruit hydrating, healing, and spiritually powerful. Archaeological evidence places watermelon seeds in the tombs of Egyptian pharaohs, believed to provide nourishment in the afterlife. These seeds date back over 5,000 years, proving that watermelon has long been a vital part of African life, not just sustenance but a source of sacred energy.

In the Kalahari Desert, wild watermelons still grow today. Indigenous African communities used these fruits to survive dry seasons, extracting hydration from the flesh and even the rind. The fruit traveled north to Egypt, then east to India, and eventually made its way to Europe and the Americas. But let's not forget: the fruit's first roots were planted in African soil.

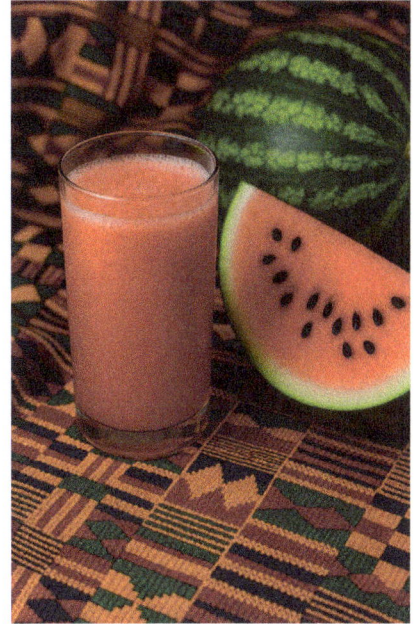

During the transatlantic slave trade, enslaved Africans brought seeds, techniques, and memories of watermelon cultivation to the Americas. In the southern U.S., Black agricultural knowledge helped watermelon flourish in plantations and gardens, though the fruit's meaning was twisted into racist caricatures by those who feared Black joy and independence. This painful history has led to generational silence, shame, or disconnection from a fruit that is truly ours.

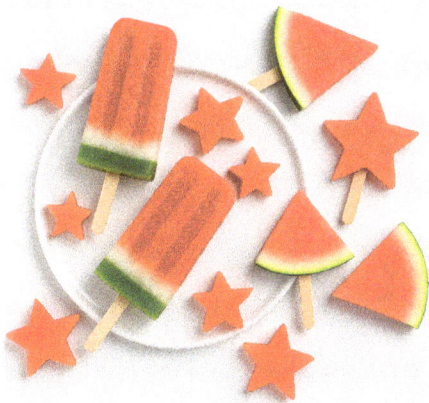

Watermelon is not just a snack. It is a symbol. It's the sweetness of survival. It's hydration in the heat of oppression. It's healing from generations of labor and loss. It is culture carved into the flesh.

Today, reclaiming the seeded watermelon bold, wild, juicy, and whole is an act of power. It means choosing the full version of yourself over the watered-down. It means honoring what was buried in soil and in history.

Let every bite you take remind you: this fruit is your inheritance.

Chapter 2: Thick & Juicy

Nutritional Benefits that Nourish You Deep

Watermelon is more than water and sugar. It's a hydrating powerhouse with nutrients that are especially beneficial for melanin-rich skin, textured hair, and Black wellness overall.

Here's why watermelon should be on every plate:

- **92% Water** – The ultimate hydration fruit, perfect for replenishing the body, improving circulation, and maintaining healthy skin tone, especially in warmer climates.

- **Vitamin A** – Supports eye health and boosts melanin production, which helps protect your skin from sun damage and aging.

- **Vitamin C** – Brightens skin, boosts immunity, and helps the body absorb iron— particularly helpful for people of African descent, who are more prone to iron deficiency.

- **Lycopene** – A powerful antioxidant that gives red watermelon its color and helps prevent chronic disease, especially heart disease and certain cancers. It's also great for skin elasticity and collagen repair.

- **Citrulline** – An amino acid found in watermelon that helps with muscle recovery and blood flow—ideal for active bodies and post-workout fuel.

- **Magnesium & Potassium** – Found in the black seeds, these minerals help regulate blood pressure, improve nerve function, and support natural hair growth from the inside out.

- **Fiber** – Watermelon supports gut health, which is directly connected to immunity, mood, and even clearer skin.

Let's not forget: the naturally occurring sugars in watermelon are balanced by its water content, making it a low-calorie snack that doesn't spike your blood sugar the way processed sweets do.

Melanin Bonus: The high-water content helps prevent ashiness and dryness from the inside out. So the next time you're sipping melon juice or munching a slice, remember you're not just snacking. You're glowing up.
Watermelon gives life.

Chapter 3: Grow Girl, Grow!

How to Grow & Pick the Right Watermelon

Want to grow your own melon? Start with the right soil: loose, sandy, and warm. Watermelon loves heat and sun. Space is key these vines like to stretch!

Planting Tips:
- Sow seeds directly after the last frost.
- Water deeply once a week.
- Harvest 75-90 days later.

How to Pick a Ripe Watermelon at the Store or Farmstand:
- Look for a creamy yellow spot (not white)
- Tap it hollow = juicy
- It should feel heavy for its size
- Skin should be dull, not shiny

Your perfect melon is waiting.

Chapter 4: Red, Yellow, Orange—Taste the Rainbow

Exploring Flesh Colors & What They Mean

Watermelon isn't one-size-flavor-fits-all. Each color comes with its own personality, history, and hidden superpowers. From sunburst orange to honey gold, *here's the juicy truth behind the rainbow of melons:*

- **Red:** The OG. This is what most people think of when they hear "watermelon." Rich in lycopene, a powerful antioxidant that supports heart health and protects the skin from sun damage. Originating in Africa and widely cultivated around the world, red watermelon is the most popular globally. Fun fact: The deeper the red, the higher the lycopene content.

- **Yellow:** The sweet surprise. Yellow watermelons are naturally sweeter and have a honey-like, almost floral taste. They're lower in lycopene but still packed with beta-carotene, which helps with eye health and immune support. Originating in Africa as a wild variant, yellow watermelon is one of the oldest flesh types recorded in historical texts.

- **Orange:** A tropical twist. With notes of mango and citrus, orange-flesh watermelon is less common but gaining attention among gourmet chefs. It contains beta-cryptoxanthin, a lesser-known antioxidant linked to joint and bone health. Some orange melons trace back to specialty farms and heirloom cultivars that value flavor over mass yield.

- **White/Pale**: The quiet ancestor. These heirloom melons are less sweet and have a crisp, cucumber-like bite. They may look underwhelming, but they're deeply hydrating and often used in traditional pickling methods across African and Asian cultures. White-flesh melons also contain trace minerals that help restore electrolyte balance.

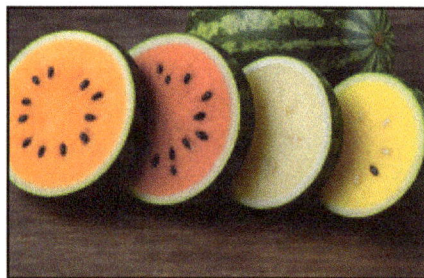

Each variety holds cultural value and nutritional depth. From red's classic heart-helping power to orange's exotic flair, and yellow's sunshine sweetness to white's ancestral crisp there's a reason to fall in love with every shade.

So don't box your melon in. Slice, sample, and celebrate the spectrum.

Chapter 5: Don't Play with Your Food—Unless It's This Cute"

Kid-Friendly Shapes, Snacks & Silliness

Melon balls, star cutouts, wacky kabobs—watermelon fun for the little ones.

Introducing picky eaters to healthy foods can feel like a challenge but watermelon? That's your secret weapon. Sweet, hydrating, colorful, and fun to cut into shapes, watermelon is the ultimate gateway fruit for kids.

Why Watermelon Works for Kids:

*   Naturally sweet without added sugars
*   Soft and easy to chew
*   Packed with hydration (great for summer days)
*   Bright colors that draw attention Safe, especially when cut into fun-sized bites

Fun Ways to Serve It:

*   **Melon Balls** – Use a melon baller to scoop bite-sized spheres. Chill them for a refreshing treat. Frozen Bites – Freeze small cubes for a teething treat or summer pops.
*   **Star, Heart & Animal Shapes** – Use cookie cutters to create magical melon moments. Kids love choosing their own shapes.
*   **Rainbow Skewers** – Alternate red, yellow, and orange melon chunks with grapes, strawberries, and pineapple on a kid-safe skewer.

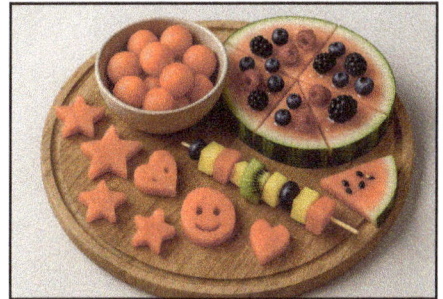

*   **Melon Pizza** – Slice a round wheel of watermelon, layer it with yogurt "sauce," berries, and a drizzle of honey. Let your little ones decorate their own slice.
*   **Juicy Cubes + Dip** – Pair watermelon cubes with a fun dip like vanilla yogurt or whipped cream and cinnamon for a make-your-own snack tray.

Hydration Hack for Parents: Got a kid who "forgets" to drink water? Give them a bowl of cold melon instead. It hydrates and satisfies—and it's easier than begging them to drink a glass.

Teen Bonus: For older kids and teens who can't seem to let go of sodas or sweet drinks, watermelon juice is the perfect replacement. It's naturally sweet, refreshing, and provides hydration without the sugar crash. Serve it chilled with mint and lime for a fun, fizzy feel or mix it with sparkling water for a soda-style sip.

Watermelon is joy in a rind. So get creative, make it cute, and let snack time double as playtime. Hydration just became the highlight of their day

Chapter 6: The Seeded Truth

Why Black Seeds Are a Gift, Not a Nuisance

For years, we've been fooled to believe that seedless watermelons are superior, cleaner, easier, and more convenient. Here's the real deal: black seeds are soulful, nutrient-packed powerhouses. They're not just part of tradition, they're part of your healing.

Black-Seeded vs. Seedless: What's the Difference?

Black-Seeded Watermelon: This is the original, natural watermelon. The seeds are mature, fertile, and edible rich in protein, magnesium, zinc, and iron. They can be roasted like pumpkin seeds or added to smoothies for a nutrient boost.

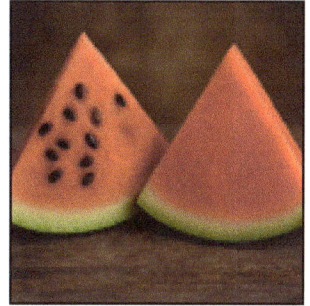

Seedless Watermelon: These are hybrid fruits created by crossing two different watermelon types to produce sterile fruit. While convenient, they're often less flavorful and lack the same nutritional value in their underdeveloped white seeds.

Nutritional Benefits of Black Seeds:

Magnesium: Essential for nerve function, muscle recovery, and energy production.
Zinc: Supports immunity and skin health.
Iron: Vital for red blood cell production—especially important in communities where iron deficiency is common.

Good Fats: Black watermelon seeds contain healthy fatty acids, which support heart and brain health.

Fertility, Folklore & Legacy:
In many African and diasporic traditions, seeds represent life, fertility, and continuation. Swallowing seeds wasn't just harmless, it was often seen as symbolic of growth. Grandmothers used to say, *"Don't spit out the blessing."* Those black seeds were a part of our nourishment and our rituals.

The Commercial Push for Seedless:
Seedless watermelon took off in the 1990s, largely due to supermarket trends and consumer convenience. What we gained in aesthetics, we lost in authenticity. Seedless varieties are often genetically manipulated and grown more for looks than legacy.

The Bottom Line:
Seedless may be trendy, but seeded is traditional, and in our world, tradition matters. Black seeds are flavorful, functional, and filled with nutrients. They're not a hassle, they're the heartbeat of the fruit.
So next time you slice open a melon, don't be afraid of those little black seeds. Roast them, blend them, or swallow them whole. Just know you're consuming culture, legacy, and strength.

Spoiler alert: Seeds are soul.

Chapter 7: Slay & Hydrate

Infused Waters & Hydration Rituals

Hydration is more than a health tip, it's a ritual, a glow-up from the inside out. And watermelon? She's the queen of the hydration throne. Whether it's hot outside or the middle of winter with dry skin knocking at your door, watermelon keeps you nourished, refreshed, and radiant.

How Our Ancestors Used It:

In ancient African traditions, watermelon was more than refreshment, it was survival. During dry seasons and long journeys, families relied on the hydration power of watermelon flesh and even its rinds. It was carried across deserts, offered during rituals, and consumed during recovery from heat exhaustion. It wasn't uncommon for grandmothers to make cooling tonics from watermelon and herbs, passing down both hydration and heritage in every sip.

All-Year Watermelon-Infused Drinks:

1. Cucumber Watermelon Cooler (Summer Refresh)
- 1 cup diced watermelon
- 1/2 cucumber, sliced
- 5 mint leaves
- 1 quart cold water

Let it infuse for 1–2 hours in the fridge. Serve with ice and a lime wedge.

2. Winter Glow Tonic
- 1 cup watermelon juice
- 1 inch fresh ginger, grated
- 1/2 lemon, squeezed
- Warm water to top off

This warms the body, boosts immunity, and keeps winter dehydration away.

3. Sparkling Melon Refresher
- **1/2 cup watermelon juice**
- **Sparkling water**
- **A splash of lime juice**
- **Optional: basil or rosemary sprig**

Perfect for replacing soda and creating a fizz without the guilt.

4. Watermelon Rose Elixir
Watermelon Rose Elixir
- 1 cup watermelon juice
- 1 tsp rose water
- Crushed ice
- Mint to garnish

It's hydrating, fragrant, and feels like a spa in a glass.

Make It a Ritual:
Start your day with a hydration moment. Before coffee or breakfast, pour yourself a glass of infused water or fresh juice. Sit quietly. Sip with intention. Let your body wake up and say thank you.

Hydration doesn't have to be boring. When you slay from the inside, the glow shows up on the outside.

Watermelon is your year-round hydration partner.
Infuse it. Blend it. Sip it. Let it heal you.

Chapter 8: Smoothie Operator

Blended Goodness from Sunrise to Sunset

Smoothies are where health meets flavor, and watermelon is the MVP of your blender. Naturally sweet, hydrating, and rich in antioxidants, watermelon blends beautifully with other fruits, veggies, and boosters to fuel your body from the inside out.

Whether you're rushing out the door, resetting after a workout, or just vibing in the kitchen, these watermelon-based smoothies will keep you glowing morning to night.

Top 5 Watermelon Smoothies:

1. Glow Up Green
For skin, energy, and natural radiance.

- 1 cup watermelon cubes
- 1/2 banana
- 1/2 cup spinach
- 1/2 cucumber
- 1/2 cup coconut water
- Squeeze of lime

Blend and feel that glow hit different.

2. Hydration Hero
The ultimate refresh after a workout or long day.

- 1 1/2 cups watermelon
- 1/2 cup strawberries
- A pinch of sea salt
- 1/2 lemon, squeezed
- 1/2 cup water or coconut water

Keeps you quenched and charged.

3. Skin So Soft
For that dewy, nourished look.

- 1 cup watermelon
- 1/2 avocado
- 1/2 cup oat milk
- 1 tablespoon flaxseed
- Dash of cinnamon

Your skin will thank you.

4. Morning Melon Fuel
A breakfast blend that powers your hustle.

- 1 cup watermelon
- 1/2 banana
- 1 tablespoon almond butter
- 1/2 cup plain Greek yogurt or dairy-free yogurt
- Handful of oats
- Splash of almond milk

Great on-the-go energy without the crash.

5. Sunset Sip
Calm your day with a cooling treat.

- 1 cup frozen watermelon cubes
- 1/2 cup pineapple
- Small piece of ginger
- 1/2 cup chamomile tea (cooled)
- Ice as needed

Unwind and let the day melt away.

Smoothie Tip: Skip the protein powder and collagen if that's not your vibe. Instead, try natural boosters like soursop, baobab fruit powder, or a spoon of soaked chia seeds. These ancestral ingredients are rich in antioxidants, fiber, and skin-loving nutrients that enhance your glow and immunity naturally.

From sunrise hustle to sunset chill, watermelon keeps you smooth, strong, and satisfied.
Now blend, sip, and slay!

Chapter 9: Juice Game Strong

Fresh Pressed Juice Recipes for Every Mood

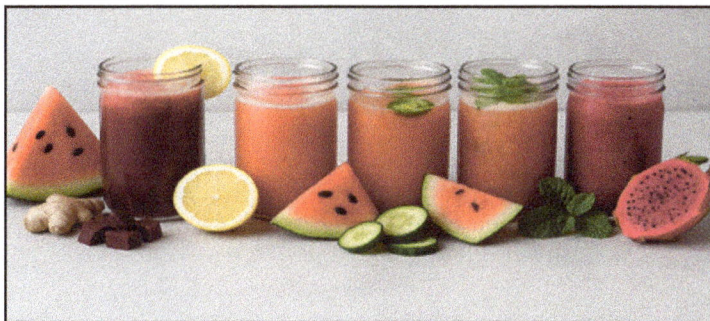

Watermelon makes the perfect base for vibrant, vitamin-packed juices that you can sip morning, noon, and night. It's naturally hydrating, gently sweet, and pairs beautifully with fruits, herbs, and spices. Whether you're cooling off, cleansing, or boosting your mood, there's juice for that.

Signature Juice Blends:

1. Beet the Heat
A bold, earthy blend packed with nutrients and glow-power.
- 1 cup watermelon
- 1/2 cup raw or roasted beets (peeled and chopped)
- Juice of 1/2 lemon
- 1/2 inch fresh ginger
- Optional: small apple or orange for sweetness

This deep red juice is rich in iron, folate, and antioxidants—perfect for circulation, cleansing, and keeping your energy steady.

2. Ginger Zing
For immunity and a little kick to your day.
- 2 cups watermelon
- 1 inch fresh ginger
- 1/2 lemon, peeled
- 4 fresh mint leaves

Juice together and serve over ice.

3. Spicy Melon Mule
For when you want bold with a bite.
- 1 1/2 cups watermelon
- 1/4 jalapeño (seeds removed)
- 1/2 cucumber
- Juice of 1 lime
- Optional: splash of sparkling water

Sweet. Spicy. Unforgettable.

4. Melon Mint Refresher
Perfect for hot days or post-workout resets.
- 2 cups watermelon
- Handful of mint leaves
- 1/2 lime, squeezed
- 1/2 cup coconut water

Blend or juice, then strain if needed. Serve chilled.

5. Dragon Glow Elixir
Antioxidant-rich and deeply hydrating.
- 1 cup watermelon
- 1/2 cup red dragon fruit
- Juice of 1 orange
- 1/2 teaspoon baobab powder (optional)

A vibrant magenta drink to help you shine from within.

6. Soursop Sunset
Smooth, tropical, and full of anti-inflammatory benefits.
- 1 cup watermelon
- 1/2 cup ripe soursop pulp (seeds removed)
- Juice of 1/2 lemon
- Dash of cinnamon or turmeric

Blend until smooth. Chill and sip slowly.

Juice Tip:
Don't toss the pulp—freeze it in ice cube trays for smoothies or use it in fruit-based dressings.
These juices aren't just drinks—they're **wellness in a glass.**
From a kick of ginger to the elegance of dragon fruit, these blends keep your juice game strong and your spirit even stronger. **Drink up!**

Chapter 10: Shake That Rind

Creative Ways to Use the Rind Don't Toss It!

In the South, nothing went to waste and watermelon rind was no exception. While the pink flesh got all the love, our ancestors knew the real prize was just beneath the surface. Watermelon rind was pickled, stewed, sautéed, and even preserved as jam. It was how they turned scraps into soul food.

Why Use the Rind?

- It's rich in citrulline, which supports blood flow and reduces inflammation.
- It's full of fiber, great for digestion.
- It's crunchy, mild, and perfect for absorbing flavor.

Ancestral Southern Rind Recipes:

1. Pickled Watermelon Rind
Sweet, tangy, and old-school.

- 4 cups watermelon rind (green skin removed, white part cubed)
- 1 cup apple cider vinegar
- 1/2 cup water
- 1/2 cup sugar or maple syrup
- 1 tbsp mustard seeds, 1 tsp cloves, 1 cinnamon stick Simmer until rinds are tender but crisp. Cool, jar, and refrigerate.

2. Southern Rind Stew
A savory side passed down in cast-iron tradition.
- 2 cups diced rind
- 1/2 onion, chopped
- 1 bell pepper, chopped
- Garlic, herbs, and vegetable broth Sauté aromatics, add rind, and simmer in broth until tender. Serve hot over rice or cornbread.

3. Rind Slaw
Bright and crunchy with a Southern twist.
- 2 cups shredded rind
- 1/2 cup shredded carrots
- 1/4 cup mayo or vegan mayo
- Apple cider vinegar, a dash of hot sauce, honey, and celery seed Chill and serve with BBQ or fried catfish.

4. Rind Jam or Preserve
Spread on toast or biscuits, just like Grandma did.

- Simmer diced rind with sugar, lemon juice, and ginger until thickened
- Blend if smoother texture is preferred

Tips from the Ancestors:
- Always peel off the outer green skin before cooking the rind.
- Add spices like clove, cinnamon, and ginger to bring out flavor.
- Cook with intention turns what was discarded into something cherished.

In Southern kitchens, watermelon rind was more than a leftover; it was a sign of resourcefulness, pride, and love. Shake that rind and honor the wisdom that never let anything go to waste.

Chapter 11: Melon Me, Please

Grilled & Savory Dishes That Surprise

When it comes to grilling, most folks think ribs, burgers, or maybe a little corn on the cob. But what if I told you that watermelon yes, sweet, juicy watermelon can step up to the grill like a Southern belle with smoky swagger?

Grilled watermelon is the ultimate curveball. The heat intensifies its sweetness while adding a bold, meaty texture that shocks and delights the taste buds. Whether you're hosting a cookout, brunching with your besties, or just tired of the same ol' sides, these recipes will have your guests saying, "Wait this is watermelon!"

Grilled Watermelon Staples
1. Watermelon Steaks with Balsamic Glaze
Savory, smoky, and totally satisfying.

- Thick watermelon slices (about 1 inch)
- Olive oil, sea salt, black pepper
- Balsamic reduction (drizzle after grilling)

Grill 2–3 minutes per side for that perfect char. Top with herbs or vegan feta for extra flair.

2. Southern BBQ Melon Sliders
A playful twist on pulled pork minus the pork.

- Grilled watermelon cubes
- Brioche or cornbread slider buns
- Rind slaw (see Chapter 10)
- Chipotle mayo or BBQ drizzle

It's a conversation piece and a crowd-pleaser in every bite.

3. Grilled Melon & Veggie Skewers
Farm stand meets the backyard grill.
- Chunks of watermelon, zucchini, bell peppers, red onion
- Brushed with olive oil, garlic powder, smoked paprika

Grill until veggies are tender and watermelon has caramelized grill marks. Pair with herbed couscous.

4. Charred Watermelon & Feta Salad
Southern heat meets Mediterranean chill.
- Grilled watermelon cubes
- Crumbled feta (or dairy-free alt)
- Fresh mint, arugula, thinly sliced red onions
- Honey-lime vinaigrette or lemon dressing

It's refreshing, sophisticated, and summer in a bowl.

5. Watermelon & Grilled Okra Bowl
A soulful bite rooted in the South.
- Grilled watermelon and okra
- Raw corn kernels
- Cherry tomatoes
- Apple cider vinaigrette
- Toasted sunflower seeds for crunch

This bowl is colorful, comforting, and nutrient-packed.

Southern Grilling Tip:
Let the grill kiss the watermelon not drown it in flames. You want seared, not soggy. Think bold edges, juicy hearts.

Grilled watermelon isn't a gimmick, it's a revolution. It's proof that with the right spice and a little smoke, our favorite fruit can cross into savory territory and still steal the show.

So go ahead, add a little fire to your fruit. Because watermelon just got grown, sexy, and grilled to perfection.

Chapter 12: Soul Sips

Watermelon-Based Drinks Inspired by the South

Some drinks aren't just beverages, they're stories in a glass. Inspired by Southern roots, Sunday porch swings, and Big Mama's backyard garden, these watermelon blends bring soul, comfort, and a touch of nostalgia with every sip.
Soul-Inspired Sips:

1. Porch Pop Watermelon Lemonade
Old-school flavor with a modern twist.

- 2 cups watermelon juice
- Juice of 2 lemons
- 1 tbsp agave or honey (optional)
- Fresh mint and lemon slices

Serve chilled over crushed ice. Add a splash of sparkling water to bring it to life.

2. Southern Sunset Tea
Melon meets sweet tea magic.

- 1 cup watermelon juice
- 1 cup cold black tea
- A splash of peach juice or puree
- Garnish with mint and orange peel

Perfect for family cookouts or solo front-porch healing.

3. Soul Shine Cooler
Hydration meets heritage.

- 1 cup watermelon
- 1/2 cup hibiscus tea (cooled)
- Squeeze of lime
- 1 tsp maple syrup or date syrup
- Crushed ice

This vibrant red drink is packed with antioxidants, Southern flair, and spiritual warmth.

4. Watermelon Bourbon Blessing (Adult Only)

- 1/2 cup watermelon juice
- 1 shot of bourbon
- A dash of smoked paprika or cayenne
- Squeeze of lime

Shake with ice and serve in a chilled glass for a soulful evening sip.
These soul sips are more than drinks, they're cultural recipes. Blend them, share them, and let them carry stories from one generation to the next.

Chapter 13: Sip Happens

Watermelon Cocktails & Adult Sips

Time to elevate your grown & sexy vibes. Whether you're hosting a rooftop mixer, cozying up for a night in, or toasting under summer stars, watermelon makes the perfect base for cocktails that are as fresh as they are flirty. Think bold flavors, vibrant colors, and a splash of soul.

Signature Watermelon Cocktails:

1. Watermelon Breeze (Malibu Twist)
Island vibes with a juicy watermelon upgrade.

- 1 oz Malibu rum (or other coconut rum)
- 2 oz watermelon juice
- 1 oz pineapple juice
- 1/2 oz lime juice
- Crushed ice
- Garnish: watermelon wedge + shredded coconut rim (optional)

Shake with ice, pour into a chilled glass, and transport yourself to your own tropical paradise.

2. Watermelon Margarita
Bold, zesty, and perfect for parties.

- 2 oz tequila
- 1 oz triple sec
- 1 oz fresh lime juice
- 3 oz watermelon juice
- Salt or Tajín rim (optional) Shake with ice and serve with a wedge of lime and a watermelon slice.

3. Melon Mojito
Minty-fresh with a mellow twist.
- 2 oz white rum
- 1 oz lime juice
- 1 oz watermelon juice
- Fresh mint, muddled
- Sparkling water to top Serve in a tall glass with crushed ice.

4. Spiked Sangria Rosé
Summery and sassy.

- 1 bottle chilled rosé wine
- 1/2 cup watermelon cubes
- 1/4 cup strawberries
- 1/4 cup pineapple
- 1/2 orange, sliced
- 1/4 cup brandy or peach schnapps Chill for 2+ hours. Serve over ice and enjoy the glow.

5. Watermelon Mimosa
Bougie brunch in a glass.

- 2 oz watermelon juice
- 4 oz chilled prosecco or champagne
- Mint sprig or melon ball garnish Light, fizzy, and Instagram-ready.

6. Melon Mule
A southern twist on a Moscow Mule.

- 2 oz vodka
- 1 oz lime juice
- 3 oz watermelon juice
- Top with ginger beer Serve in a copper mug with crushed ice and a mint sprig.

7. Honey Hush Lemon Drop

Smooth, sweet, and with just the right kick.

- 1.5 oz vodka
- 1 oz watermelon juice
- 1/2 oz lemon juice
- 1/2 oz honey or agave syrup Shake well with ice and strain into a sugar-rimmed martini glass.

Grown Folks Tip:

Make it a vibe. Add a playlist, light a candle, serve with a slice and toast to your juicy life. These cocktails aren't just for drinking, they're for celebrating the soft, bold, and beautiful version of you.

Cheers to good health and even better flavor!

Chapter 14: Cool It Down- Beat the Heat

Frozen Treats & Sorbets that Chill You Out

Sometimes you don't need heat, you need to chill. Watermelon's naturally sweet, hydrating, and freezer-friendly qualities make it the perfect base for frozen snacks that cool you from the inside out. From creamy scoops to icy pops, these recipes bring the breeze to your body and soul.

Frozen Favorites:

1. Watermelon Granita
An easy, elegant Italian-style ice.

- **4 cups watermelon, blended and strained**
- **Juice of 1 lime**
- **2 tablespoons agave or honey (optional)**

Instructions:
Pour into a shallow dish, freeze for 1 hour, then scrape with a fork every 30 minutes until fluffy. Serve in glasses with mint.

2. Juicy Ice Pops
Kid-tested, adult-approved.

- 2 cups watermelon
- 1/2 cup coconut milk or almond milk
- A splash of vanilla
- Optional: blueberries or kiwi slices added to molds

Instructions:
Blend all ingredients and freeze in popsicle molds. Great for hydration and summer fun.

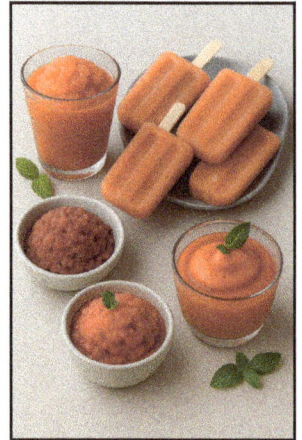

3. Melon Berry Froyo (Dairy-Free)
Creamy and tart with a watermelon twist.

- 2 cups frozen watermelon chunks
- 1 cup frozen mixed berries
- 1/2 cup plain non-dairy yogurt
- 1 tbsp maple syrup or agave

Instructions:
Blend until smooth and serve soft-serve style, or freeze for 1 hour for a scoopable texture.

4. Watermelon Sorbet
Refined, refreshing, and ridiculously simple.

- 3 cups frozen watermelon cubes
- Juice of 1/2 lemon
- Small handful of mint leaves
- 1 tbsp honey (optional)

Instructions:
Blend until smooth and creamy. Garnish with mint and enjoy immediately.

5. Sweet Heat Melon Slushie
A grown-up treat with a spicy kick.

- 2 cups frozen watermelon
- 1/4 tsp cayenne or chili powder
- Juice of 1 lime
- Splash of pineapple juice

Instructions:
Blend, sip, and feel the sweet-spicy chill roll through.

Cool Down Tip:

Freeze leftover watermelon juice in ice cube trays. Use it in smoothies, juice blends, or cocktails when you need a splash of chill.

Whether you're beating the heat or just craving something cold and clean, these treats are here to cool you down mind, body, and flavor.

Chapter 15: Sweet on You

Desserts with Heart & Hydration

Who said dessert can't be juicy and nourishing? Watermelon isn't just for snacking, it's a soulful base for sweet treats that satisfy without the sugar crash. Whether you're serving the family, treating your inner child, or celebrating a special moment, these watermelon-based desserts offer cooling comfort with every bite.

Sweet Favorites:

1. Watermelon Shortcake
Southern charm meets juicy delight.

- Watermelon rounds or thick slices in place of cake
- Fresh whipped cream or coconut cream
- Macerated strawberries or blackberries
- Layer and serve like traditional shortcake for a light, refreshing twist

2. Honey-Drizzled Watermelon Cubes
Simple, elegant, unforgettable.

- Chilled watermelon cubes
- Light drizzle of raw honey
- Sprinkle of cinnamon
- Garnish with mint or edible flowers Perfect for summer gatherings or quick afternoon indulgence.

3. Watermelon Cupcakes (Mini Melon Muffins)
Fun, moist, and family friendly.

- Blend watermelon into cupcake batter (pairs great with vanilla or lemon)
- Add chocolate chips or a cream cheese swirl
- Frost with whipped topping or yogurt icing Moisture from the melon gives these bakes a soft, juicy crumb.

4. Vegan Melon Tart
Fresh, fruity, and no-bake fabulous.

- Crust: dates, almonds, and coconut pressed into a tart pan
- Filling: blended watermelon and soaked cashews with a splash of lemon
- Top with kiwi slices, berries, and mint Chill until firm and serve cold.

5. Frozen Watermelon Bites with Dark Chocolate
Decadent meets hydrating.

- Freeze watermelon cubes
- Dip halfway into melted dark chocolate
- Sprinkle with crushed pistachios or sea salt Keep frozen until ready to serve.

Dessert Tip:

Watermelon's natural moisture means less added sugar and fat. When crafting desserts, lean into its freshness, add a squeeze of citrus or pair with bold spices like cardamom or ginger to elevate the experience.

These sweets are more than just treats; they're tender moments, joyful bites, and a little slice of juicy love. ***You deserve it.***

Chapter 16: Brunch Goals

Melon-Infused Breakfast Recipes

Rise and shine the watermelon way. Brunch is your chance to slow down, nourish intentionally, and serve up joy whether it's Sunday morning or just a much-needed reset. Watermelon brings freshness, color, and gentle sweetness to every plate. It's brunch that hydrates, heals, and hits the soul.

Morning Favorites:

1. Watermelon Toast with Whipped Feta Crisp, creamy, and cool.

- Whole grain or sourdough toast
- Whipped feta (blend feta with Greek yogurt or vegan alternative)
- Thin watermelon slices
- Drizzle of honey or balsamic glaze
- Garnish with fresh mint and cracked pepper Perfect for a savory-sweet start.

2. Melon & Berry Breakfast Parfait Layers of love.

- Chopped watermelon
- Mixed berries (blueberries, raspberries, strawberries)
- Greek or coconut yogurt
- Granola or chia pudding Layer in a glass jar for a beautiful, portable power breakfast.

3. Watermelon Pancakes with Mint Syrup Pillowy goodness with a melon twist.

- Pancake batter (add a splash of blended watermelon to the mix)
- Cook as usual, then top with chopped watermelon and a mint-infused maple syrup (heat maple syrup with fresh mint leaves and strain) Optional: sprinkle of lime zest.

4. Melon Sunrise Smoothie Bowl Bright, bold, and beautiful.

- Smoothie base: blended watermelon, frozen mango, banana
- Toppings: shredded coconut, pumpkin seeds, chia, and melon balls Scoop and sparkle with every bite.

5. Watermelon Breakfast Salsa A refreshing topper for eggs, toast, or avocado.

- Diced watermelon
- Diced avocado
- Red onion, lime juice, cilantro, pinch of salt Serve over scrambled eggs or grain bowls for a zesty start.

Brunch Tip:

Make it a vibe, set the table with sliced melon, colorful plates, and herbal tea. Brunch isn't just about the food, it's about savoring the slow moments.
Start the day juicy. ***You deserve it.***

Chapter 17: Date Night, Done Right

Elegant Recipes with Watermelon Flair

A romantic night deserves more than takeout; it deserves thoughtfulness, flavor, and maybe just a little flirtation on the fork. Watermelon, with its bold sweetness and refreshing nature, can bring elegance and charm to any dinner date. Whether you're cooking for someone special or celebrating yourself, these watermelon-inspired dishes are sensual, simple, and undeniably swoon-worthy.

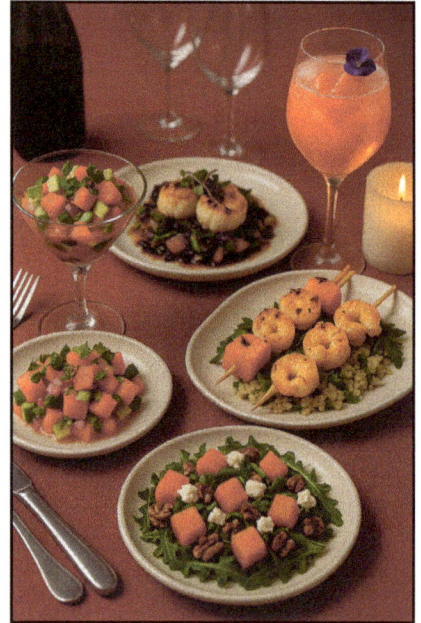

Love-Infused Recipes:

1. Watermelon Ceviche
Light, zesty, and bursting with freshness.
- Diced watermelon
- Diced avocado
- Chopped red onion
- Jalapeño (optional, for heat)
- Fresh lime juice
- Cilantro and sea salt

Instructions:
Chill and serve in a martini glass or on endive leaves for a refined, plant-based twist on classic ceviche.

2. Seared Scallops over Melon Slaw
Sea-meets-sweet in a perfect bite.
- Pan-seared scallops (3–5 per person)
- Watermelon rind and cabbage slaw
  (with vinegar, honey, and mint dressing)
- Garnish: microgreens and a drizzle of balsamic glaze

Instructions:
Elegant, colorful, and full of texture.

3. Watermelon & Goat Cheese Arugula Salad
Bittersweet balance made for romance.
- Cubed watermelon
- Crumbled goat cheese
- Fresh arugula
- Candied pecans or walnuts
- Light lemon vinaigrette

Instructions:
Serve with wine and candlelight for extra charm.

4. Grilled Shrimp and Melon Skewers
Savory, smoky, and sensual.
- Large shrimp, peeled and deveined
- Watermelon chunks
- Olive oil, garlic, and lime zest

Instructions:
Brush shrimp and melon with seasoning. Grill until just charred and serve with herbed couscous. This dish looks like art and tastes like love.

5. Candle-Lit Watermelon Spritz
A toast to slow love.
- 2 oz watermelon juice
- 2 oz elderflower liqueur (or sparkling rosé)
- 1/2 oz lemon juice
- Sparkling water to top
- Garnish: edible flower or frozen melon cube

Instructions:
Serve chilled in your favorite glass. Sip slowly and savor the moment.

Date Night Tip:
Cook together. Laugh at the mess. Feed each other bites.
Whether you're dating, married, or solo and glowing, let this meal remind you:
Love like watermelon is best served fresh and full of flavor.

Chapter 18: Glow Up, Gorgeous

Watermelon Beauty Hacks & Skincare Secrets

Watermelon isn't just good for your body, it's a whole glow-up for your skin. From ancient cooling rituals to modern spa hacks, this fruit is packed with vitamins, antioxidants, and hydration that give your skin the love it deserves.

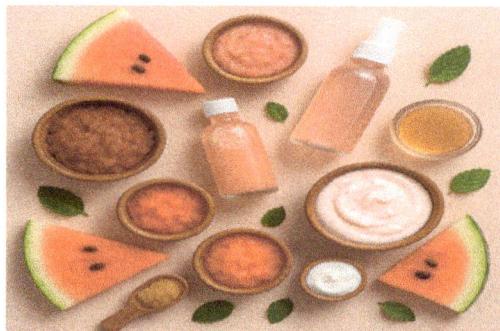

DIY Beauty Recipes:

1. Watermelon Toner Refreshes, tightens, and brightens.

- 1/2 cup watermelon juice (strained)
- 1 tbsp rose water
- Optional: 1 tsp witch hazel (for oily skin) Dab on with a cotton round or mist on after cleansing. Keep refrigerated for up to 5 days.

2. Glow-Up Face Mask For soft, hydrated skin.

- 2 tbsp mashed watermelon
- 1 tbsp plain Greek yogurt or aloe vera gel
- 1 tsp honey Apply to clean skin for 10–15 minutes, rinse with cool water, and pat dry. Use 2x a week.

3. After-Sun Cooling Spray Soothes sun-kissed or irritated skin.

- 1/2 cup watermelon juice
- 1/4 cup cucumber juice
- 1 tsp aloe vera juice Store in a spray bottle and mist your face or body for instant cooling and hydration.

4. Watermelon Sugar Scrub Buff away dry skin, hello glow.

- 1/2 cup watermelon pulp
- 1/2 cup brown sugar
- 1 tbsp coconut oil Scrub in gentle circles on arms, legs, or back. Rinse well. Smells divine and leaves skin silky.

5. Lip Plump & Polish Soft lips with a hint of shine.

- 1 tbsp watermelon juice
- 1 tsp sugar
- 1/2 tsp shea butter or coconut oil Gently rub onto lips, then wipe away for a smooth, kissable pout.

Beauty Tip:

Store your beauty blends in the fridge for extra freshness. Always patch test before full use, especially if you have sensitive skin.

Let your skincare feel sacred. Let your self-care be sweet. You don't need a spa just a slice of watermelon and the time to glow.

Chapter 19: Detox Like a Queen

Meal Prep & Clean Eating with Watermelon as Your Base

Watermelon isn't just a treat, it's a detox dream. With its high water content, natural sweetness, and nutritional power, watermelon helps flush out toxins, support digestion, and keep you full without the bloat. This chapter shows you how to build a clean-eating week around melon magic.

Why Detox with Watermelon?

- Naturally diuretic and anti-inflammatory
- Hydrates while satisfying sweet cravings
- Pairs well with veggies, grains, and healthy fats
- Light on the stomach and easy to digest

Mindful Melon Meal Ideas:

1. Daily Detox Bowl

- Base: arugula or kale
- Toppings: watermelon cubes, avocado slices, cucumber, sunflower seeds
- Dressing: lemon + olive oil + a pinch of cayenne Perfect for lunch that keeps you light and energized.

2. Watermelon & Quinoa Power Jar

- Layer cooked quinoa, watermelon chunks, black beans, red onion, and lime juice in a mason jar
- Shake and eat on-the-go Make-ahead friendly and packed with fiber and protein.

3. Green Glow Wraps

- Romaine or collard leaves
- Fill with shredded carrots, grilled watermelon strips, and hummus or avocado mash
- Roll tight and enjoy fresh raw, crunchy snack or light lunch.

4. Post-Cleanse Watermelon Soup

- Blend watermelon with mint, lime juice, and a pinch of sea salt
- Chill and serve as a hydrating side or sipable snack Great after a long day or a fast.

5. Sweet-Savory Snack Box

- Sliced watermelon, cucumber sticks, cherry tomatoes, olives, and hummus
- Pack in bento boxes for mid-morning or late-day snacking Balanced. Beautiful. Bite-sized.

Weekly Prep Tip:

Cut and cube a large watermelon at the start of the week. Store in airtight containers and use it daily for smoothies, salads, infused waters, and quick snacks. Keep a jar of dressing and prepped greens nearby for instant meal magic.

Cleansing doesn't mean restricting. With watermelon at the center, detox becomes delicious, nourishing, and sustainable just the way a queen deserves.

Chapter 20: Melon for the Culture

Soul Food Remix — Watermelon in Black Cuisine

It's time to take back the narrative. Watermelon, long used as a tool for harmful stereotypes, has deep, sacred roots in Black culinary history. This chapter is about reclaiming that truth. With reverence and flavor, we remix watermelon into soul food recipes that are full of love, dignity, and joy.

Addressing the Myth:

Let's be clear: there's nothing shameful about loving good southern fried chicken and cooling off with sweet hydration watermelon. Both were staples of survival and celebration in our communities. The shame came from racist depictions, not from the food itself. It's time to remove that stigma and honor the creativity and resilience of Black cooks throughout history.

Soulful Watermelon Traditions & New Classics:

1. Hot Honey Watermelon & Chicken Bites Sweet heat with a golden crunch.

- Crispy baked or air-fried chicken tenders
- Cubed watermelon tossed in hot honey, lime juice, and sea salt Serve together on skewers for a flavorful appetizer that honors both tradition and innovation.

2. Collard & Melon Wraps Fresh twist on a soul food staple.

- Use large collard leaves as wraps
- Fill with grilled watermelon, black-eyed peas, and herbed rice
- Top with tangy mustard vinaigrette This one's light, vibrant, and deeply rooted.

3. Watermelon Cornbread Bake A sweet-savory side dish remix.

- Traditional cornbread batter
- Swirl in diced watermelon and roasted jalapeños
- Bake and serve with cinnamon butter It's moist, surprising, and addictive.

4. Black-Eyed Pea & Melon Salad Good luck never tasted so fresh.

- Black-eyed peas, cubed watermelon, red onion, cilantro, and avocado
- Toss with lemon juice, olive oil, and cumin Perfect for cookouts, Juneteenth, or any celebration.

5. Fried Green Tomatoes with Watermelon Chutney Crunch, tang, and sweet all in one.

- Classic cornmeal-crusted fried green tomatoes
- Top with a quick chutney made from watermelon, vinegar, and ginger Serve warm with fresh herbs.

Cultural Cooking Tip:

As you prepare these dishes, play some soul music, speak your ancestors' names, and remember: this is how we heal. With every plate, we're rewriting the story one bite at a time.

This isn't just food. It's a reclamation. It's resistance. It's for the culture.

Chapter 21: Still Juicy – Honoring Our Ancestors

Legacy, Healing & Living Out Loud

This isn't just the end of a guide
It's the beginning of something more.
A lifestyle. A reclamation.
A soulful celebration of your **heritage, health, and healing.**

Watermelon has walked with us from **ancestral fields** to **Sunday tables**, from **backyard cookouts** to **beauty rituals.**

It has **nourished bodies, carried stories,** and **soothed spirits.**
Now, it's here to remind you of your own power.

Reflect
- What tradition do you want to reclaim or create?
- What healing did this journey stir in you?
- What joy did you taste on each page?

Ritual
End this journey with blessing...
Say a word of gratitude for your body, your ancestors, and your journey.
Take a bite with intention.
That's your **legacy**, right there.

Don't Forget Affirmations
I am rooted in something sweet and strong.
I glow from within and hydrate with purpose.
I honor my past, nourish my present, and grow toward my future.
My life is full of sweet flavor, full-filling life.

Final Word
This book isn't just about watermelon. It's about **choosing yourself**, every single day.
It's about **healing loudly, living boldly,** and never being ashamed of what feeds your **body and soul.**

www.ingramcontent.com/pod-product-compliance
Lightning Source LLC
Chambersburg PA
CBHW041601260326
41914CB00011B/1345